Retirement Eats: Delicious and Healthy Recipes for the Golden Years

Judy Kelly

Table of Contents:

Chapter 7

Meal Planning and Prep

- Meal planning tips for retirees
- How to make the most of leftovers
- How to stock a healthy pantry
- How to modify recipes for dietary restrictions

Conclusion

- Thank you for using Retirement Eats
- Additional resources for healthy eating in retirement
- Final thoughts and suggestions.

Chapter 1

Introduction

Retirement Eats: Delicious and Healthy Recipes for the Golden Years" is the ultimate cookbook for seniors who want to enjoy delicious, healthy meals while also staying active and fit. As we age, it becomes increasingly important to pay attention to our diet and make sure we're getting the nutrients we need to stay healthy and energized.

This cookbook is designed to make it easy for seniors to enjoy delicious, healthy meals without sacrificing taste or convenience. Inside, you'll find a wide variety of recipes that are easy to make, full of flavor, and packed with nutrients. From hearty breakfasts to satisfying dinners, this cookbook has something for every taste and dietary need. Whether you're looking for low-calorie, low-fat, or gluten-free options, you'll find them here. With easy-to-follow recipes and helpful tips and tricks, "Retirement Eats" is the perfect guide for seniors who want to make the most of their golden years with delicious, healthy food.

Welcome to Retirement Eats

Welcome to "Retirement Eats: Delicious and Healthy Recipes for the Golden Years"! We are thrilled to share this collection of delicious and nutritious recipes that are perfect for seniors. As we age, it becomes more important to pay attention to our diet and make sure we are getting the nutrients we need to stay healthy and energized. This cookbook is designed to make it easy for seniors to enjoy delicious, healthy meals without sacrificing taste or convenience. Inside, you will find a wide variety of recipes that are easy to make, full of flavor, and packed with nutrients. From hearty breakfasts to satisfying dinners, this cookbook has something for every taste and dietary need. Whether you are looking for low-calorie, low-fat, or gluten-free options, you will find them here. With easy-to-follow recipes and helpful tips and tricks, "Retirement Eats" is the perfect guide for seniors who want to make the most of their golden years with delicious, healthy food. So, let's get started on this culinary journey together!

How to use this cookbook

Retirement Eats: Delicious and Healthy Recipes for the Golden Years" is designed to be user-friendly and easy to follow. Here are a few tips on how to make the most out of this cookbook:

1. Browse the Table of Contents: The Table of Contents is located at the beginning of the cookbook and provides an overview of the different sections and recipes included. This is a great way to get a sense of what the cookbook has to offer and to find recipes that interest you.

2. Read the recipe's introduction: Each recipe includes an introduction that provides a brief overview of the dish, including

the ingredients and cooking time. This will help you determine if a recipe is appropriate for your skill level and dietary needs.

3. Gather ingredients: Before you start cooking, make sure you have all of the ingredients listed in the recipe. This will save you time and ensure that your dishes come out as delicious as possible.

4. Follow the instructions carefully: The instructions for each recipe are written in a step-by-step format to make them easy to follow. Be sure to read them carefully and pay attention to any special instructions or tips included.

5. Enjoy your meal: After you've followed the recipe and cooked your dish, sit down, relax, and enjoy your delicious and healthy meal. Don't forget to take a picture of your dishes and share it with your friends and family!

6. Remember that you can always adjust the recipe according to your taste and dietary needs. Cooking is an art and as you gain more experience you'll be able to personalize the recipe to your liking. We hope you enjoy using "Retirement Eats" and that it helps you to create delicious, healthy meals that you'll love. Bon Appetit!

The importance of healthy eating in retirement

Eating a healthy and balanced diet is important for people of all ages, but it is especially important for retirees. As people age, their nutritional needs change, and it is important to make sure that their diet provides the necessary nutrients to support overall health and well-being.

One of the main concerns for older adults is maintaining a healthy weight and avoiding obesity, which can lead to a host of health problems such as diabetes, heart disease, and high blood pressure. A healthy diet that includes a variety of fruits, vegetables, whole grains, and lean proteins can help retirees maintain a healthy weight and reduce their risk of these conditions.

Retirees also have a greater need for certain nutrients such as calcium and vitamin D to support bone health. Eating a diet rich in these nutrients can help prevent osteoporosis and reduce the risk of fractures.

In addition, retirees may also be at a higher risk of certain health conditions such as constipation, which can be prevented or managed by incorporating foods high in fiber into their diet.

Eating a healthy and balanced diet can also improve overall energy levels, and mental clarity and promote a sense of well-being.

Overall, healthy eating is an essential part of maintaining good health in retirement and can help retirees stay active and independent for as long as possible.

Chapter 2

Breakfast Recipes

Oatmeal Breakfast Bars

Ingredients:

2 cups rolled oats

1 cup whole wheat flour

1/2 cup chopped nuts (walnuts, almonds, pecans, etc.)

1/2 cup dried fruit (raisins, cranberries, apricots, etc.)

1/2 cup honey

1/4 cup coconut oil

1 egg

1 tsp vanilla extract

1/2 tsp baking powder

1/4 tsp salt

Instructions:

1. Preheat your oven to 350°F (175°C). Grease an 8x8-inch baking dish with cooking spray.
2. In a large bowl, combine the oats, flour, nuts, and dried fruit.
3. In a separate bowl, whisk together the honey, coconut oil, egg, vanilla extract, baking powder, and salt.

4. Pour the wet ingredients into the dry ingredients and stir until everything is well combined.

5. Press the mixture evenly into the prepared baking dish.

6. Bake for 20-25 minutes or until the edges are golden brown.

7. Let the bars cool in the baking dish for 10 minutes, then transfer them to a wire rack to cool completely.

8. Once the bars have cooled, cut them into squares or bars and enjoy.

These oatmeal breakfast bars are a great option for a grab-and-go breakfast or a healthy snack. They are also easy to make and you can customize the recipe by adding different kinds of nuts and dried fruits to your taste. You can store the bars in an airtight container at room temperature for up to a week.

Vegetable Frittata

Ingredients:

8 eggs

1/2 cup milk

1/4 tsp salt

1/4 tsp black pepper

2 tbsp olive oil

1 small onion, chopped

1 red bell pepper, diced

1 cup cherry tomatoes, halved

1 cup spinach, chopped

1/4 cup grated Parmesan cheese (optional)

Instructions:

1. Preheat the oven to 350°F (175°C).
2. In a large bowl, whisk together the eggs, milk, salt, and pepper.
3. In a large oven-safe skillet, heat the olive oil over medium heat. Add the onion and bell pepper and cook until softened, about 5 minutes.
4. Add the cherry tomatoes and spinach to the skillet and cook until the spinach is wilted about 2 minutes.

5. Pour the egg mixture into the skillet and stir gently to combine with the vegetables. Cook for 2-3 minutes, or until the edges start to set.

6. Sprinkle the Parmesan cheese over the top of the frittata, if using.

7. Transfer the skillet to the oven and bake for 15-20 minutes, or until the frittata is set and the top is golden brown.

8. Remove the skillet from the oven and let it cool for a few minutes.

9. Use a spatula to carefully slide the frittata out of the skillet onto a cutting board.

10. Cut the frittata into wedges and serve warm or at room temperature.

This is a great recipe that you can customize with any vegetables you have on hand. You can also add some diced cooked potatoes or sweet potatoes to make it more filling. You can serve it with a side of greens or a salad for a balanced meal. You can enjoy the leftovers for lunch or dinner the next day.

Breakfast recipes

Berry and Yogurt Smoothie Bowl

Ingredients:

1 cup frozen mixed berries (strawberries, blueberries, raspberries, blackberries)

1/2 banana

1/2 cup Greek yogurt

1/2 cup milk or milk alternative

1 tsp honey (optional)

Toppings: chopped nuts, seeds, granola, coconut flakes, fresh berries

Instructions:

1. In a blender, combine the frozen berries, banana, Greek yogurt, milk or milk alternative, and honey, if using.
2. Blend on high speed until smooth and creamy. If the mixture is too thick, add a bit more milk or a milk alternative to reach the desired consistency.
3. Pour the smoothie into a bowl.
4. Add your toppings of choice, like chopped nuts, seeds, granola, coconut flakes, and fresh berries.

Enjoy your smoothie bowl immediately!

This recipe is a delicious and healthy breakfast option that you can customize to your taste, you can add any kind of fruits you like, or even add some spinach or kale to boost the nutrients. You can also play with the toppings, adding different kinds of nuts, seeds, granola, and fruits. This smoothie bowl is a great way to start your day with a boost of energy and vitamins.

Breakfast recipes

Yoghurt Parfait with Granola

Ingredients:

1 cup Greek yogurt

1/4 cup granola

1/4 cup fresh berries (strawberries, blueberries, raspberries)

1 tbsp honey (optional)

Instructions:

1. In a jar or a bowl, layer the Greek yogurt, granola, and berries.
2. Drizzle with honey, if desired.
3. Repeat the layering process until you reach the top of the jar or bowl.
4. Cover the jar or bowl with a lid or plastic wrap and refrigerate for at least 30 minutes.
5. Before serving, give the jar or bowl a gentle shake or stir to distribute the granola evenly.

Enjoy your parfait!

This is a simple and delicious recipe that you can customize according to your preferences. You can use any type of yogurt and add different kinds of fruits and nuts to your liking. You can also use different kinds of granola, like gluten-free, low-sugar, or homemade granola. The parfait can be made ahead of time and kept in the fridge, this way you can have a healthy breakfast ready in the morning.

Breakfast recipes

Blueberry muffins

Ingredients:

2 cups all-purpose flour

1/2 cup granulated sugar

2 tsp baking powder

1/2 tsp salt

1/2 cup unsalted butter, melted and cooled

2 large eggs

1/2 cup milk

1 tsp vanilla extract

1 cup fresh blueberries

Instructions:

1. Preheat the oven to 375°F (190°C). Line a 12-cup muffin tin with paper liners.
2. In a large mixing bowl, whisk together the flour, sugar, baking powder, and salt.
3. In a separate bowl, whisk together the melted butter, eggs, milk, and vanilla extract.
4. Pour the wet ingredients into the dry ingredients and stir until just combined.
5. Gently fold in the blueberries.

6. Using a spoon or a cookie scoop, divide the batter evenly among the muffin cups.

7. Bake the muffins for 20-25 minutes or until a toothpick inserted into the center of a muffin comes out clean.

8. Remove the muffins from the oven and let them cool in the tin for 5 minutes.

9. Take the muffins out of the tin and transfer them to a wire rack to cool completely.

These blueberry muffins are perfect for a quick breakfast on the go or as a snack. They can be stored in an airtight container at room temperature for up to 3 days, or in the refrigerator for up to 5 days. You can also freeze the muffins for up to 3 months. To thaw, place the frozen muffins on a plate and let them sit at room temperature for 30 minutes before serving.

Chapter 3

Salads and Appetizers

Greek Salad

Ingredients:

1 large cucumber, diced

1-pint cherry tomatoes, halved

1/2 red onion, thinly sliced

1/2 cup kalamata olives, pitted

1/2 cup crumbled feta cheese

1/4 cup chopped fresh parsley

2 tbsp extra-virgin olive oil

2 tbsp red wine vinegar

1 clove garlic, minced

Salt and pepper to taste

Instructions:

1. In a large bowl, combine the cucumber, tomatoes, red onion, olives, feta cheese, and parsley
2. In a small bowl, whisk together the olive oil, red wine vinegar, garlic, salt, and pepper.
3. Pour the dressing over the salad and toss to coat evenly.

4. Serve immediately or refrigerate for at least 30 minutes before serving to allow the flavors to meld together.

This is a classic Greek salad recipe that is perfect for a light and refreshing lunch or dinner. You can add some diced cooked chicken or shrimp to make it more filling. The salad can be served as a side dish or as a main dish. The best way to enjoy this salad is with some nice fresh bread to sop up the delicious dressing.

Salads and Appetizers

Caesar Salad

Ingredients:

1 head of romaine lettuce, washed and chopped

1/2 cup croutons

1/4 cup grated Parmesan cheese

2 cloves of garlic, minced

1/4 cup mayonnaise

2 tablespoons fresh lemon juice

2 tablespoons Dijon mustard

2 tablespoons Worcestershire sauce

1/4 cup extra-virgin olive oil

Salt and pepper to taste

Instructions:

1. In a large bowl, combine the chopped romaine lettuce, croutons, and grated Parmesan cheese.
2. In a small bowl, whisk together the garlic, mayonnaise, lemon juice, Dijon mustard, Worcestershire sauce, olive oil, salt and pepper.
3. Pour the dressing over the salad and toss to coat evenly.
4. Serve immediately or refrigerate for at least 30 minutes before serving to allow the flavors to meld together.

This is a classic Caesar salad recipe that is perfect for a light and refreshing lunch or dinner. You can add some grilled chicken or shrimp to make it more filling. The salad can be served as a side dish or as a main dish. You can also add some anchovies or capers for extra flavor. The best way to enjoy this salad is with some fresh crusty bread to sop up the delicious dressing.

Caprese Salad

Ingredients:

2-3 large ripe tomatoes, sliced

8 oz fresh mozzarella cheese, sliced

1/4 cup fresh basil leaves

2-3 tablespoons extra-virgin olive oil

Salt and pepper to taste

Balsamic glaze (optional)

Instructions:

1. Arrange the tomato slices on a serving platter or individual plates.
2. Top with the slices of mozzarella cheese.
3. Scatter the basil leaves over the tomatoes and cheese.
4. Drizzle the olive oil over the salad and season with salt and pepper to taste.
5. If desired, drizzle balsamic glaze over the salad.

Serve immediately and enjoy!

This is a classic Caprese salad recipe that is perfect for a light and refreshing lunch or dinner. It is a simple and delicious salad that showcases the freshness and flavor of the ingredients. The combination of the sweet and juicy tomatoes, creamy mozzarella cheese and fragrant basil leaves makes this salad irresistible. The balsamic glaze is optional, but it adds a nice sweet and tangy note to the salad. This salad can be served as a side dish or as a main dish.

Salad and Appetizers

Shrimp Cocktail

Ingredients:

1 lb raw shrimp, peeled and deveined

1/4 cup lemon juice

2 cloves garlic, minced

1 tbsp Worcestershire sauce

1 tbsp hot sauce

2 tbsp ketchup

1/4 cup chopped fresh cilantro

Salt and pepper to taste

Lemon wedges and cocktail sauce for serving

Instructions:

1. Bring a large pot of water to a boil. Add the shrimp and cook for 2-3 minutes or until they turn pink and are fully cooked. Drain and rinse the shrimp with cold water.

2. In a large bowl, whisk together the lemon juice, garlic, Worcestershire sauce, hot sauce, ketchup, cilantro, salt, and pepper.

3. Add the shrimp to the bowl and toss to coat evenly with the marinade.

4. Cover the bowl with plastic wrap and refrigerate for at least 30 minutes or up to 2 hours to allow the flavors to meld together.

5. To serve, arrange the shrimp on a platter and garnish with lemon wedges and cilantro. Serve with cocktail sauce on the side.

This shrimp cocktail recipe is a classic and delicious appetizer that is perfect for entertaining. The shrimp are cooked in a flavorful marinade made with lemon juice, garlic, Worcestershire sauce, hot sauce and ketchup. The shrimp can be served cold or at room temperature, with a classic cocktail sauce or with a spicy sauce. This recipe is easy to prepare and can be made ahead

Baked Brie with Cranberry Sauce

Ingredients:

1 wheel of brie cheese

1/2 cup cranberry sauce

1/4 cup chopped pecans or walnuts

1 tbsp honey

Puff pastry (store-bought or homemade)

1 egg, beaten

Instructions:

1. Preheat the oven to 375°F (190°C).
2. Roll out the puff pastry on a lightly floured surface to a thickness of about 1/8 inch.
3. Place the brie cheese in the center of the puff pastry.
4. Spread the cranberry sauce over the top of the brie.
5. Sprinkle the chopped pecans or walnuts over the cranberry sauce.
6. Drizzle the honey over the nuts.
7. Fold the puff pastry up and around the brie, making sure to completely enclose it.
8. Brush the beaten egg over the pastry.

9. Place the wrapped brie on a baking sheet and bake for 20-25 minutes or until the pastry is golden brown and puffed.

10.   Let the brie cool for 5 minutes before slicing and serving.

This Baked Brie with Cranberry Sauce is a classic and delicious appetizer that is perfect for entertaining. The combination of the creamy brie cheese and the sweet and tangy cranberry sauce is irresistible. The nuts and honey add a nice crunch and sweetness to the dish. The puff pastry adds a nice flaky texture.

Chapter 4

Main Dishes

Lemon Herb Chicken

Ingredients:

4 boneless, skinless chicken breasts

Salt and pepper

1/4 cup all-purpose flour

2 tablespoons olive oil

2 cloves garlic, minced

1/4 cup chicken broth

1/4 cup fresh lemon juice

2 tablespoons butter

2 tablespoons chopped fresh parsley

2 tablespoons chopped fresh thyme

Instructions:

1. Season the chicken breasts with salt and pepper. Dredge the chicken in the flour.
2. In a large skillet, heat the olive oil over medium-high heat. Add the chicken and cook until golden brown on both sides, about 5 minutes per side. Remove the chicken from the skillet and set aside.

3. Add the garlic to the skillet and cook for 1 minute.

4. Add the chicken broth and lemon juice to the skillet and bring to a boil.

5. Reduce the heat to medium-low and add the butter. Whisk until the butter is melted and the sauce is emulsified.

6. Return the chicken to the skillet and spoon the sauce over the chicken.

7. Sprinkle the parsley and thyme over the chicken.

8. Cover the skillet and simmer for 10-15 minutes or until the chicken is cooked through.

9. Remove the skillet from the heat and let it sit for 5 minutes.

10. Serve the chicken with the sauce spooned over the top.

This Lemon Herb Chicken recipe is a classic and delicious dish that is perfect for a weeknight dinner. The combination of the lemon juice and herbs adds a nice fresh and fragrant flavor to the dish. You can serve the chicken with a side of pasta, rice or vegetables to make a complete meal. This recipe is easy to make, but it is packed with flavor.

Grilled Fish with Mango Salsa

Ingredients:

4 (6-ounce) fish fillets (such as salmon, halibut, or cod)

Salt and pepper

1 tbsp olive oil

1/4 tsp cumin

1/4 tsp chili powder

1/4 tsp paprika

1/4 tsp garlic powder

1 mango, peeled and diced

1/4 red onion, diced

1/4 red bell pepper, diced

2 tbsp chopped fresh cilantro

2 tbsp lime juice

Instructions:

1. Season the fish fillets with salt and pepper.
2. In a small bowl, whisk together the olive oil, cumin, chili powder, paprika and garlic powder. Brush the mixture over the fish fillets.
3. Preheat the grill to medium-high heat. Grill the fish for 4-6 minutes per side, or until it is cooked through and flakes easily with a fork.

4. While the fish is grilling, make the salsa by mixing together the diced mango, red onion, red bell pepper, cilantro and lime juice in a medium bowl. Season with salt and pepper to taste.

5. Remove the fish from the grill and serve with the mango salsa on top or on the side.

This Grilled Fish with Mango Salsa Recipe is a delicious and healthy dish that is perfect for summertime grilling. The fish is seasoned with a flavorful spice rub and grilled to perfection, while the mango salsa adds a sweet and refreshing contrast. The mango salsa is easy to make and can be prepared ahead of time. The combination of flavors is absolutely delicious. The salsa can also be used as a topping for grilled chicken or pork. This recipe is easy to make and it is a great way to enjoy fish, it's a perfect dish for a summer dinner.

Main Dishes

Slow cooker beef stew

Ingredients:

1 lb beef chuck roast, cut into 1-inch cubes

2 cups beef broth

1 cup red wine

1 onion, chopped

2 cloves of garlic, minced

2 carrots, peeled and chopped

2 stalks celery, chopped

1 lb small red potatoes, halved

1 tbsp tomato paste

2 tsp dried thyme

1 tsp dried rosemary

1 bay leaf

Salt and pepper to taste

Instructions:

1. Season the beef cubes with salt and pepper.
2. In a large skillet, heat a tablespoon of oil over medium-high heat. Add the beef cubes and cook until browned on all sides.
3. Transfer the beef to a slow cooker.
4. In the same skillet, sauté the onion and garlic until softened.

5. Add the beef broth, red wine, tomato paste, thyme, rosemary, and bay leaf to the skillet. Bring to a simmer and scrape up any browned bits from the bottom of the pan.

6. Pour the mixture over the beef in the slow cooker.

7. Add the carrots, celery, and potatoes to the slow cooker.

8. Stir everything to combine and season with salt and pepper to taste.

9. Cover the slow cooker and cook on low for 8 hours or on high for 4 hours, or until the beef and vegetables are tender.

10. Discard the bay leaf and ladle the stew into bowls.

This Slow Cooker Beef Stew recipe is a classic and comforting dish that is perfect for cold winter days. The beef is cooked to tender perfection in a rich and flavorful broth made with red wine, beef broth, and herbs. The vegetables add a nice balance of flavors and textures to the dish. This recipe is easy to make, you just need to brown the beef and sauté the onion and garlic before adding everything to the slow cooker. You can serve the stew with some crusty bread to soak up the delicious gravy.

Vegetable lasagna

Ingredients:

1 lb lasagna noodles

1 tbsp olive oil

1 onion, chopped

2 cloves of garlic, minced

1 zucchini, sliced

1 yellow squash, sliced

1 red bell pepper, sliced

1 eggplant, sliced

2 cups marinara sauce

2 cups ricotta cheese

1 cup grated mozzarella cheese

1/4 cup grated Parmesan cheese

2 tbsp chopped fresh basil

Salt and pepper to taste

Instructions:

1. Preheat the oven to 375°F (190°C).
2. Cook the lasagna noodles according to the package instructions. Drain and set aside.

3. In a large skillet, heat the olive oil over medium heat. Add the onion and garlic and sauté until softened.

4. Add the zucchini, yellow squash, red bell pepper, and eggplant to the skillet. Sauté for about 8-10 minutes or until vegetables are tender.

5. Season with salt and pepper to taste.

6. In a large bowl, mix together the ricotta cheese, 1/2 cup mozzarella cheese, 1/4 cup Parmesan cheese, and basil.

7. Spread 1 cup of marinara sauce in the bottom of a 9x13 inch baking dish.

8. Layer 3-4 lasagna noodles over the sauce. Spread 1/3 of the ricotta mixture over the noodles. Top with 1/3 of the vegetable mixture.

Quinoa and Black Bean Enchiladas

Ingredients:

1 cup quinoa, cooked according to package instructions

1 can black beans, drained and rinsed

1/2 red onion, diced

1 red bell pepper, diced

2 cloves of garlic, minced

2 cups enchilada sauce (store-bought or homemade)

1 cup shredded cheddar cheese

8-10 corn tortillas

Fresh cilantro, diced tomatoes or avocado for topping (optional)

Instructions:

1. Preheat the oven to 375°F (190°C).
2. In a large bowl, mix together the cooked quinoa, black beans, red onion, red bell pepper, garlic, 1 cup of enchilada sauce, and 1/2 cup of shredded cheese.
3. Spread about 1/4 cup of enchilada sauce on the bottom of a 9x13 inch baking dish.
4. Warm the tortillas in a dry skillet over medium heat for about 30 seconds on each side or until they are soft and pliable.

5. Fill each tortilla with about 1/4 cup of the quinoa mixture and roll it up tightly.

6. Place the enchiladas seam-side down in the baking dish.

7. Top the enchiladas with the remaining enchilada sauce and shredded cheese.

8. Bake for 20-25 minutes or until the cheese is melted and the enchiladas are heated through.

9. Let the enchiladas cool for 5 minutes before serving. Garnish with cilantro, diced tomatoes, or avocado if desired.

This Quinoa and Black Bean Enchiladas recipe is a delicious and healthy alternative to traditional beef or chicken enchiladas. The quinoa and black beans provide a good source of protein, while the vegetables add a nice balance of flavors and textures. The enchilada sauce can be store-bought or homemade, you can use your favorite one. The tortillas can be replaced with gluten-free tortillas if needed. This recipe is easy to make and it is perfect for a weeknight dinner, you can also make them ahead of time and reheat them for a quick meal.

Chapter 5

Sides and Snacks

Roasted Brussels Sprouts with Pecans

Ingredients:

1 lb Brussels sprouts, trimmed and halved

2 tbsp olive oil

Salt and pepper

1/4 cup chopped pecans

2 tbsp maple syrup

2 tbsp balsamic vinegar

Instructions:

Preheat the oven to 425°F (220°C).

1. In a large bowl, toss the Brussels sprouts with olive oil, salt, and pepper.
2. Spread the Brussels sprouts out on a baking sheet in a single layer.
3. Roast for 20-25 minutes or until the Brussels sprouts are golden brown and tender.
4. While the Brussels sprouts are roasting, toast the pecans in a dry skillet over medium heat for about 2-3 minutes or until fragrant.
5. In a small bowl, whisk together the maple syrup and balsamic vinegar.

6. Once the Brussels sprouts are done roasting, remove them from the oven and toss them with the pecans and maple balsamic glaze. Serve immediately and enjoy.

This Roasted Brussels Sprouts with Pecans recipe is a delicious and easy side dish that is perfect for a weeknight dinner. The Brussels sprouts are roasted to perfection and the pecans add a nice crunch and sweetness to the dish. The maple balsamic glaze adds a nice sweetness and tanginess to the dish. This recipe is easy to make and it is a great way to enjoy Brussels sprouts. You can also add some bacon or prosciutto for extra flavor.

Grilled Eggplant and Zucchini

Ingredients:

1 eggplant, sliced

1 zucchini, sliced

3 tbsp olive oil

2 cloves of garlic, minced

2 tbsp balsamic vinegar

1 tsp dried oregano

Salt and pepper to taste

Instructions:

1. Preheat the grill to medium-high heat.
2. In a large bowl, mix together the olive oil, garlic, balsamic vinegar, oregano, salt and pepper.
3. Add the eggplant and zucchini to the bowl and toss to coat evenly.
4. Place the eggplant and zucchini slices on the grill and cook for about 3-4 minutes per side or until they are tender and grill marks appear.
5. Remove the eggplant and zucchini from the grill and place them on a platter.
6. Sprinkle with additional salt and pepper if desired.

Serve warm and enjoy! This Grilled Eggplant and Zucchini recipe is a delicious and healthy side dish that is perfect for a summer barbecue. The eggplant and zucchini are marinated in a flavorful mixture of olive oil, garlic, balsamic vinegar, and oregano before being grilled to perfection. The eggplant and zucchini become tender with a nice smoky flavor after being grilled. This recipe is easy to make and it's a great way to enjoy

Crispy Baked Sweet Potato Fries

Ingredients:

2 large sweet potatoes, peeled and cut into fries

2 tbsp olive oil

1 tsp paprika

1 tsp garlic powder

1 tsp salt

1/2 tsp black pepper

Instructions:

1. Preheat the oven to 425°F (220°C).
2. In a large bowl, toss the sweet potato fries with olive oil, paprika, garlic powder, salt, and black pepper.
3. Arrange the fries on a baking sheet in a single layer.
4. Bake the fries for 20-25 minutes or until they are crispy and golden brown, flipping them halfway through.
5. Remove the fries from the oven and season with additional salt if desired.

Serve immediately and enjoy!

This Crispy Baked Sweet Potato Fries recipe is a delicious and healthy alternative to traditional french fries. The sweet potatoes are cut into fries, seasoned with a mixture of spices, and baked to perfection. The result is a crispy and flavorful fry that is perfect for a side dish or a snack. This recipe is easy to make and it's a great way to enjoy sweet potatoes. You can also add some herbs like rosemary or thyme for extra flavor.

Homemade Trail Mix

Ingredients:

1 cup roasted almonds

1 cup roasted cashews

1 cup dried cranberries

1 cup dried apricots

1 cup pumpkin seeds

1 cup dark chocolate chips

Instructions:

1. In a large bowl, mix together the almonds, cashews, cranberries, apricots, pumpkin seeds, and dark chocolate chips.

2. Store the trail mix in an airtight container or resealable bag at room temperature for up to 2 weeks.

3. Enjoy as a snack, or pack some in a bag to take with you on the go.

This Homemade Trail Mix recipe is a delicious and healthy snack that is perfect for on the go. You can use your favorite nuts and dried fruits to make this trail mix. You can also change the ratio of nuts, dried fruits and chocolate chip according to your preference. This recipe is easy to make and it's a great way to enjoy a healthy and tasty snack. You can also add some seeds like sunflower seeds, flax seeds or sesame seeds for extra nutrition.

Whole wheat crackers

Ingredients:

1 cup whole wheat flour

1/2 cup all-purpose flour

1/2 tsp salt

1/4 tsp black pepper

1/4 cup olive oil

1/4 cup water

Additional seasonings of your choice (such as sesame seeds, herbs, or spices)

Instructions:

1. In a large bowl, mix together the whole wheat flour, all-purpose flour, salt, pepper, and any additional seasonings you desire.
2. Add the olive oil and water, and stir until a dough forms.
3. Knead the dough for a few minutes until smooth.
4. Roll out the dough on a lightly floured surface to 1/8 inch thickness.
5. Cut the dough into desired cracker shapes using a knife or a pizza cutter.
6. Place the crackers on a baking sheet lined with parchment paper.

7. Bake in a preheated 350°F (175°C) oven for 15-20 minutes or until golden brown.

8. Remove from the oven and let cool on a wire rack.

Store in an airtight container for up to a week.

This Whole Wheat Crackers recipe is a delicious and healthy alternative to store-bought crackers. The crackers are made with whole wheat flour and are seasoned with salt, pepper and additional seasonings of your choice. The crackers can be cut into different shape and size. This recipe is easy to make and it's a great way to enjoy a healthy and tasty snack. They are perfect with dips, cheese, or as a snack by themselves.

Chapter 6

Desserts

Chocolate Chip Cookies

Ingredients:

2 cups all-purpose flour

1 tsp baking soda

1/2 tsp salt

1/2 cup (1 stick) unsalted butter, at room temperature

1/2 cup granulated sugar

1/2 cup brown sugar

1 egg

1 tsp vanilla extract

1 cup semisweet chocolate chips

Instructions:

1. Preheat the oven to 350°F (175°C) and line a baking sheet with parchment paper.
2. In a medium bowl, mix together the flour, baking soda, and salt.
3. In a separate large bowl, cream together the butter, granulated sugar, and brown sugar using an electric mixer until light and fluffy.
4. Beat in the egg and vanilla extract until well combined.

5. Gradually add the flour mixture to the butter mixture, mixing until just combined.

6. Stir in the chocolate chips.

7. Using a cookie scoop or spoon, drop dough balls onto the prepared baking sheet.

8. Bake for 12-15 minutes or until the edges are golden brown.

9. Remove from the oven and let cool on the baking sheet for 5 minutes before transferring to a wire rack to cool completely.

This Chocolate Chip Cookies recipe is a classic and delicious treat that is perfect for any occasion. The cookies are soft and chewy on the inside and slightly crispy on the outside. The chocolate chips add a nice touch of sweetness and chocolate flavor to the cookies. You can also add nuts or dried fruits for extra flavor. This recipe is easy to make and it's a great way to enjoy a tasty and comforting cookie.

Apple Crumble

Ingredients:

Filling:

6 cups peeled, cored and thinly sliced apples

1/2 cup granulated sugar

1 tsp ground cinnamon

1/4 tsp ground nutmeg

1 tbsp lemon juice

Crumble Topping:

1 cup all-purpose flour

1/2 cup granulated sugar

1/2 cup cold unsalted butter, cut into small cubes

1 tsp ground cinnamon

1/4 tsp salt

Instructions:

1. Preheat the oven to 375°F (190°C).
2. In a large bowl, mix together the sliced apples, sugar, cinnamon, nutmeg, and lemon juice.
3. Transfer the mixture to a 9x13 inch baking dish.

4. In a separate bowl, mix together the flour, sugar, butter, cinnamon, and salt for the crumble topping.

5. Sprinkle the crumble topping evenly over the apples.

6. Bake for 40-45 minutes or until the apples are tender and the crumble is golden brown.

7. Remove from the oven and let cool for 10 minutes before serving.

Serve warm with ice cream or whipped cream, if desired.

This Apple Crumble recipe is a delicious and comforting dessert that is perfect for fall. The apples are cooked to perfection with a mixture of sugar and spices, and the crumble topping is made with flour, butter, sugar and cinnamon. The result is a sweet and crispy topping that is a perfect complement to the tender apples. This recipe is easy to make and it's a great way to enjoy apples during the fall season. You can also use a mixture of apples to give a variety of flavors and texture to the crumble.

Blueberry Cheesecake Bars

Ingredients:

Crust:

1 1/2 cups graham cracker crumbs

1/4 cup granulated sugar

1/2 cup unsalted butter, melted

Filling:

24 oz cream cheese, at room temperature

1 cup granulated sugar

4 large eggs

2 tsp vanilla extract

1 cup blueberry preserves

Instructions:

1. Preheat the oven to 325°F (165°C) and line a 9x13 inch baking dish with parchment paper.

2. In a medium bowl, mix together the graham cracker crumbs, sugar, and melted butter. Press the mixture into the bottom of the prepared baking dish.

3. In a separate large bowl, beat the cream cheese and sugar together until smooth. Beat in the eggs one at a time, then stir in the vanilla extract.

4. Pour the cream cheese mixture over the crust, spreading it evenly.

5. Drop spoonfuls of the blueberry preserves over the cream cheese mixture and swirl it in with a knife.

6. Bake for 40-45 minutes or until the edges are golden brown and the center is set.

7. Remove from the oven and let cool for 1 hour before refrigerating for at least 3 hours.

8. Cut into squares and serve chilled.

This Blueberry Cheesecake Bars recipe is a delicious and easy dessert that is perfect for any occasion. The crust is made with graham cracker crumbs, sugar, and butter. The filling is made with cream cheese, sugar, eggs and vanilla. The blueberry preserves are swirled into the cheesecake filling, which gives a nice balance of sweetness and tanginess. This recipe is easy to make and it's a great way to enjoy a cheesecake. You can also use other fruits preserves like strawberry or raspberry instead of blueberry.

Deserts

Fresh Peach Sorbet

Ingredients:

4 cups fresh peaches, peeled, pitted, and diced

3/4 cup granulated sugar

1/2 cup water

1 tbsp fresh lemon juice

Instructions:

1. In a medium saucepan, combine the peaches, sugar, and water. Bring to a boil over medium heat, then reduce the heat and simmer for about 10 minutes or until the peaches are very soft.

2. Remove from heat and let cool for 10 minutes.

3. Puree the peach mixture in a blender or food processor until smooth.

4. Strain the mixture through a fine-mesh sieve to remove any solids.

5. Stir in the lemon juice.

6. Pour the mixture into a shallow dish and freeze for about 2 hours, or until the edges begin to freeze.

7. Using a fork, scrape the frozen mixture to break up any ice crystals.

8. Freeze again for at least 4 hours, or until firm.

9. Scoop the sorbet into bowls and serve immediately.

This Fresh Peach Sorbet recipe is a delicious and refreshing dessert that is perfect for a summer day. The sorbet is made with fresh peaches, sugar, water, and lemon juice. The result is a light and flavorful sorbet that is perfect for a summer day. This recipe is easy to make and it's a great way to enjoy fresh peaches. You can also add other flavors like mint or ginger for extra flavor. Serve the sorbet in a cone, a bowl, or in a glass with a spoon, and enjoy it as a dessert or a refreshing snack.

Deserts

Chocolate Mousse

Ingredients:

8 oz bittersweet chocolate, chopped

1/2 cup heavy cream

4 large eggs, separated

1/4 cup granulated sugar

1 tsp vanilla extract

Instructions:

1. In a heatproof bowl set over a pot of simmering water, melt the chocolate and cream together, stirring until smooth. Remove from heat and let cool slightly.
2. In a large bowl, beat the egg yolks and sugar together until pale and thick. Stir in the melted chocolate mixture and vanilla extract.
3. In a separate bowl, beat the egg whites until stiff peaks form.
4. Gently fold the egg whites into the chocolate mixture until well combined.
5. Divide the mousse into serving dishes and chill for at least 2 hours or until set.
6. Serve chilled and garnish with whipped cream or berries, if desired.

This Chocolate Mousse recipe is a classic French dessert that is rich, creamy, and delicious. The mousse is made with bittersweet chocolate, heavy cream, egg yolks, sugar, and vanilla extract. The result is a creamy and decadent chocolate mousse that is perfect for any occasion. This recipe is easy to make, it's a great way to enjoy a chocolate treat, it's perfect for a dinner party or a special occasion. You can also add a tablespoon of liqueur like Grand Marnier or Chambord to give an extra flavor to the mousse.

Chapter 7

Meal Planning and Prep

When meal planning for retirees, it's important to consider their unique needs and preferences. Here are some tips for meal planning for retirees:

- Keep it simple: Simple meals that are easy to prepare and don't require a lot of ingredients are a great option for retirees. Avoid recipes that are too complicated or require a lot of cooking time.

- Plan for leftovers: Retirees may not want to cook every day, so plan for leftovers that can be easily reheated.

- Consider dietary restrictions: Many retirees may have dietary restrictions such as low-salt, low-fat, or gluten-free diets. Make sure to plan meals that are suitable for these restrictions.

- Plan for variety: While keeping meals simple, make sure to plan for a variety of different meals to keep things interesting and ensure that retirees are getting a well-balanced diet.

- Incorporate healthy ingredients: Retirees need to maintain a healthy diet as they age. Plan meals that are high in fruits, vegetables, whole grains, and lean proteins.

- Plan for the company: Retirees may enjoy having friends or family over for meals. Plan meals that can be easily shared and served in larger portions.

By taking these considerations into account, you can create a meal plan that is tailored to the unique needs and preferences of retirees and help them to maintain a healthy diet as they age.

Meal planning tips for retirees

When meal planning for retirees, it's important to consider their unique needs and preferences. Here are some tips for meal planning for retirees:

- Keep it simple: Simple meals that are easy to prepare and don't require a lot of ingredients are a great option for retirees. Avoid recipes that are too complicated or require a lot of cooking time.

- Plan for leftovers: Retirees may not want to cook every day, so plan for leftovers that can be easily reheated.

- Consider dietary restrictions: Many retirees may have dietary restrictions such as low-salt, low-fat, or gluten-free diets. Make sure to plan meals that are suitable for these restrictions.

- Plan for variety: While keeping meals simple, make sure to plan for a variety of different meals to keep things interesting and ensure that retirees are getting a well-balanced diet.

- Incorporate healthy ingredients: Retirees need to maintain a healthy diet as they age. Plan meals that are high in fruits, vegetables, whole grains, and lean proteins.

- Plan for the company: Retirees may enjoy having friends or family over for meals. Plan meals that can be easily shared and served in larger portions.

- Use a meal delivery service: Some retirees may have difficulty getting to the grocery store or preparing meals on their own. There are meal delivery services that provide pre-made, healthy meals that are easy to heat and eat.

- Make use of a slow cooker: Slow cookers can be a great tool for retirees who want to have a home-cooked meal without spending a lot of time in the kitchen.

By taking these considerations into account, you can create a meal plan that is tailored to the unique needs and preferences of retirees and help them to maintain a healthy diet as they age.

How to make the most of leftovers

Leftovers can be a great way to save time and money, but it's important to make sure they are stored and reheated properly to ensure food safety and to prevent them from going to waste. Here are some tips for making the most of leftovers:

- Store leftovers properly: Make sure to store leftovers in airtight containers and label them with the date they were made.

- Keep track of the fridge: Keep track of the food you have in the fridge and use the oldest leftovers first.

- Reheat leftovers safely: Reheat leftovers to an internal temperature of at least 165°F (74°C) to ensure that any bacteria present in the food is killed.

- Get creative: Leftovers don't have to be eaten as is, you can get creative with them, you can use leftovers to make new meals, such as a stir-fry, a sandwich, a quesadilla, a frittata, a soup, a casserole.

- Freeze leftovers: If you know you won't be able to eat leftovers within a few days, freeze them. Foods can be safely frozen for several months.

- Leftovers for lunch: Pack leftovers for lunch the next day, it's a great way to save money and ensure you have a healthy meal on hand.

By following these tips, you can make the most of your leftovers, ensure that they are safe to eat, and enjoy delicious and healthy meals throughout the week.

How to stock a healthy pantry

- Stocking a healthy pantry is an important part of maintaining a healthy diet. Here are some tips for stocking a healthy pantry:

- Whole grains: Whole grains such as quinoa, brown rice, and whole wheat pasta are a great source of fiber and nutrients.

- Canned goods: Canned goods such as beans, tomatoes, and vegetables are a great way to add nutrients to your meals.

- Nuts and seeds: Nuts and seeds such as almonds, walnuts, and chia seeds are a great source of protein and healthy fats.

- Herbs and spices: Herbs and spices such as turmeric, ginger, and cumin can add flavor and nutrition to your meals.

- Healthy oils: Healthy oils such as olive oil, avocado oil, and coconut oil are a great way to add flavor and healthy fats to your meals.

- Dried fruits: Dried fruits such as raisins, cranberries, and apricots are a great source of fiber and antioxidants.

- Protein sources: Protein sources such as canned tuna, canned salmon, and frozen chicken are a great way to add protein to your meals.

- Baking essentials: Baking essentials such as flour, sugar, and baking powder are a great way to make healthy homemade snacks and meals.

By stocking your pantry with these healthy options, you'll be able to make nutritious meals and snacks quickly and easily.

How to modify recipes for dietary restrictions

Modifying recipes for dietary restrictions can be a bit tricky, but it's definitely possible. Here are some tips for modifying recipes for dietary restrictions:

- Substitute ingredients: Substitute ingredients such as using gluten-free flour for wheat flour, almond milk for cow's milk, or avocado for butter.

- Omit ingredients: Omit ingredients such as cheese or nuts if someone has a dairy or nut allergy.

- Add alternative ingredients: If a recipe calls for a specific ingredient that is not suitable for a dietary restriction, try adding an alternative ingredient that will provide similar flavor and texture.

- Use alternative cooking methods: If a recipe calls for deep-frying, try baking or grilling instead.

- Get creative: Get creative and experiment with new ingredients and flavors to make the recipe suitable for dietary restrictions.

- Research: Research and try different recipes specifically designed for the dietary restriction, it's a great way to get inspiration and ideas.

- Seek professional help: If you have any doubts about how to modify a recipe for a specific dietary restriction, you can seek professional help from a dietitian or a nutritionist.

By following these tips, you can modify recipes to make them suitable for dietary restrictions, and still enjoy delicious and nutritious meals. Remember that when it comes to dietary restrictions, safety comes first, so make sure to consult with a doctor or a dietitian if you have any doubts.

Conclusion

Thank you for using Retire-ment Eats

Thank you for choosing to use our cookbook, "Retirement Eats: Delicious and Healthy Recipes for the Golden Years." We hope that you have enjoyed trying out the recipes and that they have helped you to maintain a healthy and delicious diet during your retirement. We hope you find the recipes easy to follow, delicious and nutritious. We are delighted that we could be a part of your cooking journey and enhance your dining experience. We appreciate your support and feedback, and we look forward to hearing about your culinary adventures. Thank you again for using our cookbook, and we wish you happy and healthy eating!

Additional resources for healthy eating in retirement

There are many resources available to help retirees maintain a healthy diet. Here are a few additional resources for healthy eating in retirement:

1. Government websites: Websites such as the USDA's MyPlate (https://www.choosemyplate.gov/) provide information on healthy eating and nutrition for older adults.

2. Dietitians and nutritionists: Consulting with a registered dietitian or nutritionist can provide personalized advice and guidance on healthy eating for retirees.

3. Senior centers: Many senior centers offer cooking classes and nutrition education programs specifically designed for older adults.

4. Online communities: There are many online communities and forums dedicated to healthy eating and nutrition for retirees.

5. Cookbooks and recipe websites: There are many cookbooks and recipe websites specifically designed for retirees, with recipes that are healthy and easy to prepare.

6. Support groups: Support groups for retirees with specific dietary restrictions, such as gluten-free or low-salt diets, can provide valuable information and support.

By utilizing these resources, retirees can access the information and support they need to maintain a healthy diet during their golden years.

Final thoughts and suggestions.

Maintaining a healthy diet during retirement is important for overall health and well-being. The cookbook "Retirement Eats: Delicious and Healthy Recipes for the Golden Years" provides a variety of easy-to-make and nutritious recipes that are tailored to the needs and preferences of retirees. By following the meal planning and preparation tips provided, retirees can easily plan and prepare healthy and delicious meals throughout the week. Additionally, making use of the additional resources such as government websites, dietitians, senior centers, and online communities can provide further support and guidance for healthy eating in retirement. Remember to listen to your body and seek professional help if you have any doubts about your diet and nutrition.

www.ingramcontent.com/pod-product-compliance
Lightning Source LLC
Chambersburg PA
CBHW081810250726
48653CB00010B/3865